waiting
on the universe

waiting on the universe
a collection of poems

Priscilla T. Brown

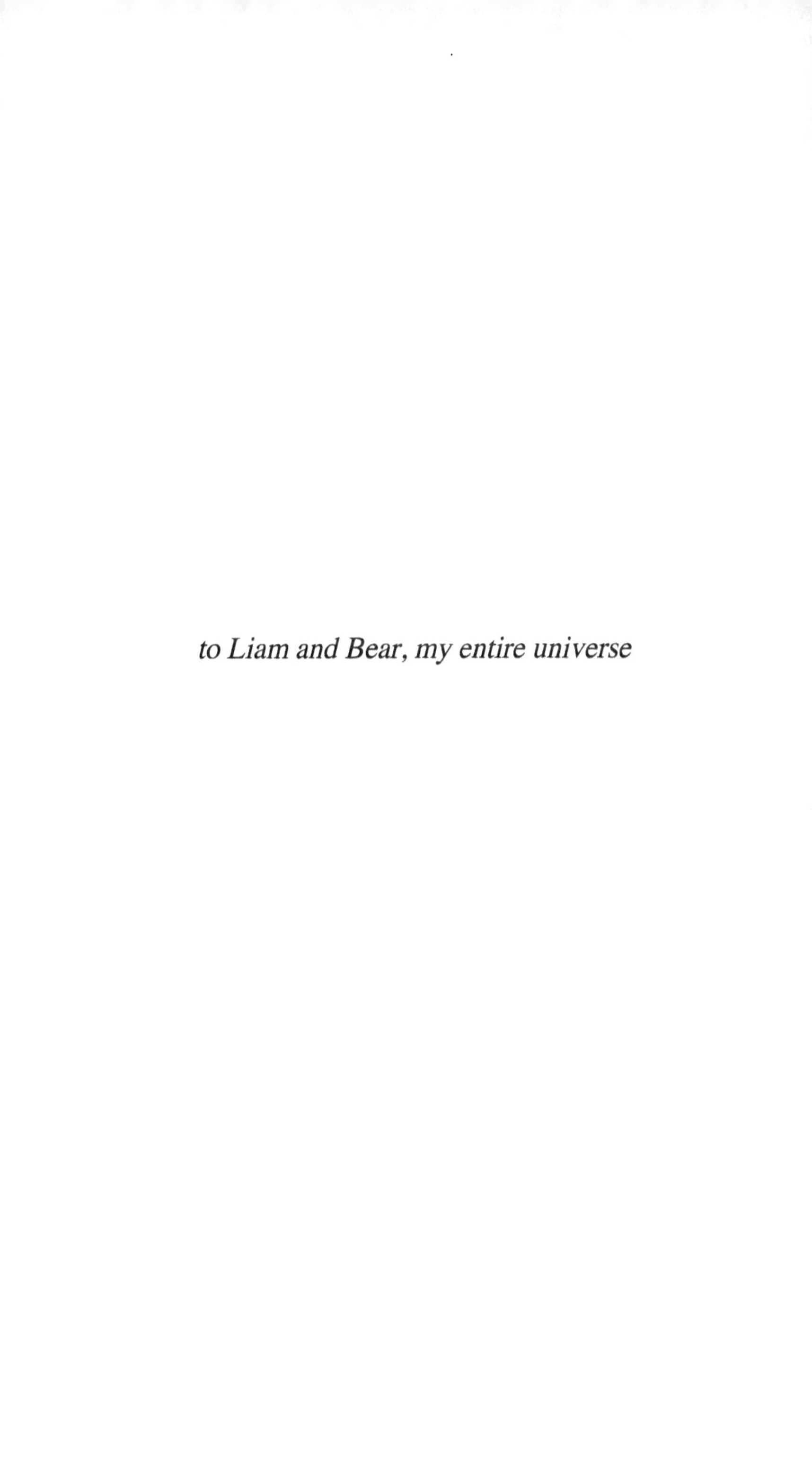

to Liam and Bear, my entire universe

contents

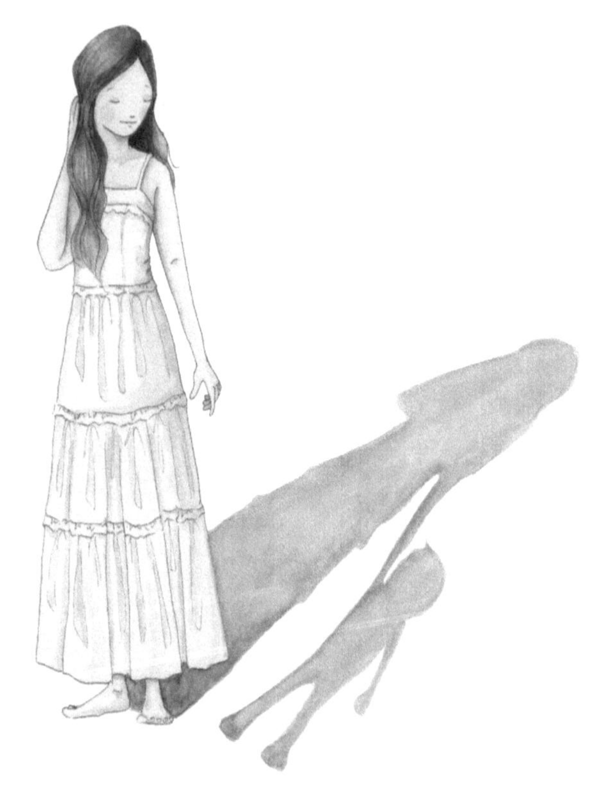

"Tell the story of the mountain you climbed.
Your words could become a page
in someone else's survival guide."
- Morgan Harper Nichols

i n t r o d u c t i o n

They told me I would never get pregnant. But then I did.
Twice. So I never bothered to ask if I could write a book.

Sometimes on the way to becoming a parent, the universe decides it has a different plan. What you thought would be an easy journey instead becomes years of pain, loss, waiting, and wondering.

waiting on the universe is a collection of letters and poems I wrote over the years to a child I wasn't certain would ever exist. Our "someday baby" that I dreamed of as we struggled to get pregnant. Writing these pages became therapeutic during the hard times and remained a big piece of my heart for many years.

I published this book so that these pages could bring hope to anyone out there who may need it; that these poems could give solace to anyone who may be grieving or stumbling through life's toughest storms; and that my words could provide support to anyone struggling to make sense of infertility.

I hope this book helps you continue fighting, wishing, dreaming, and shouting to the universe that you are worthy, you are waiting for your baby, and you are not giving up easily. And never let anyone stop your dream of becoming a parent.

xx Priscilla

chapter one: waiting

may 2012 - june 2014

Looking back at the years we struggled to get pregnant, the days were filled with music festivals, hiking trips, DIY home projects, and newlywed movie night cuddles on the couch, all while a huge elephant sat in the room. The smiles that appear in photographs show the memories I hope to remember, although buried within were moments I decisively labeled as "the worst of times."

We tried on our own to get pregnant. We did just as we were instructed to do which was to keep trying and simply wait to see what happens. At first it was fun and exciting. We were oblivious that anything was physically wrong and we were full of optimism as we anticipated starting a family. But as the weeks turned into months and then into years, we continued to wait for a pregnancy that wasn't coming.

I watched the world around us continue to breeze by like the wind. I watched as friends brought home their babies, proudly beaming from ear to ear, as I longed for it to someday be my turn. I listened as whispers of "*maybe it's not meant to be*" filled my ears and crowded my mind. I waited, not so patiently, for a sign to come. A plus sign on a plastic pregnancy stick or a grandiose response from the universe to give me some answers. I waited.

Soon the waiting turned into desperate pleas and prayers. Praying to God, the universe, a shooting star, birthday candles, dandelion pedals, pennies in a fountain, or to anyone who would listen that somewhere out there our baby was also waiting for us and that he or she was only a few sunrises away.

the tide was coming in
as we sat in our boat built for two.
rocking back and forth
floating under a hot june sky.
he hooked the bait
and i cast my line.
the sunbeams caught my skin
as i looked up at him and smiled.
sweat dripped from his brow
though he didn't seem to notice.
we quietly passed the time.
busy hands and busy hearts
fishing off the shore line
we talked
of sons and daughters
of returning here one day
in a boat built for four
or perhaps even more.
we cruised back
as the daylight fell from the sky.
and all the while
we were dreaming of you.

how could it possibly be
that in a field full of wildflowers
none grow for me?

if i were given a million wishes
        and a million dreams come true
i'd throw it all back into the sea
        if it meant i could just have you.

when you get here
    i'll be ready.

i'll teach you everything i know
    or make it up for you as we go.

we'll share laughter as we play
    inside jokes only we can say.

i'll be your comfort, your shield, your light
    the one who tucks you in bed at night.

i'll help you rise to be your best,
    i'll be the heartbeat in your chest.

when you get here
    i'll be ready.

my darling, when will you get here?
    i am ready.

some mornings i wake up from a dream,
a dream that vanishes
faster than the words can escape my mouth
leaving no memory
that it was even there.
as if the universe is begging me to forget.
yet somehow i still know
that in my dreams
          you are always there.

another day has come
the sun shines bright
but you're still not here.
if you were
i'd show you that sun.
i'd hold you on my lap
and we'd listen to the trees.
we'd wait for the moon to arrive
and i'd sing you a song.
we'd count all the stars
as you'd fall asleep in my arms.

but you are still not here.
so just as the sun waits
each morning to return,
i'll wait each day for you.

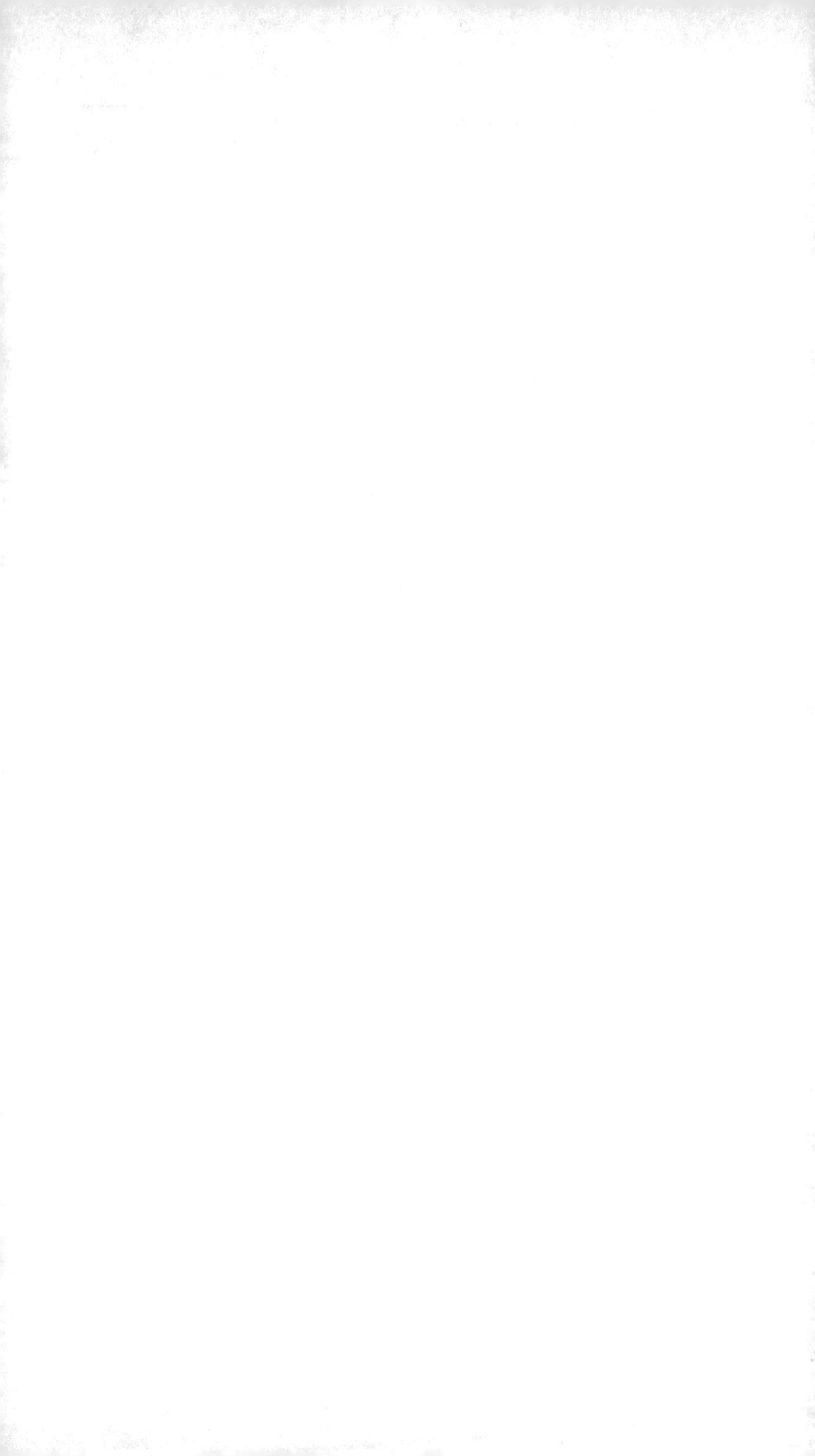

i dream of a world full of wonder.
a place where magic is real
where dreams come true
and miracles are only a sunrise away.
a world where you are here
and the universe whispers to me,
          "i did this just for you."

i don't know where you are
but standing here
underneath billions of stars
knowing how one day
they will all shine
just for you,
this simply seems
like the right place to be.

she waited for her baby
for it was all she knew to do.
if only the universe could tell her
he was out there waiting too.

just as i know the earth turns
i know you'll come to me one day.
for even in the cloudiest
darkest of nights
the sun is somewhere out there
waiting for its time to rise.

what a wonderful world
       full of things to do.
you are here now.
       and i am too.
carpool lines and lullabies.
       teddy bears and a kiss goodnight.
cotton swaddles and bubble baths,
       pajama parties and belly laughs.
go to bed, not one more peep.
       i stay awake to watch you sleep.
night after night,
       this picture of us.
i picture it…
       then i wake up.

do not sail out
into the rough seas
wait there on the shore, my love
i'll get there eventually.

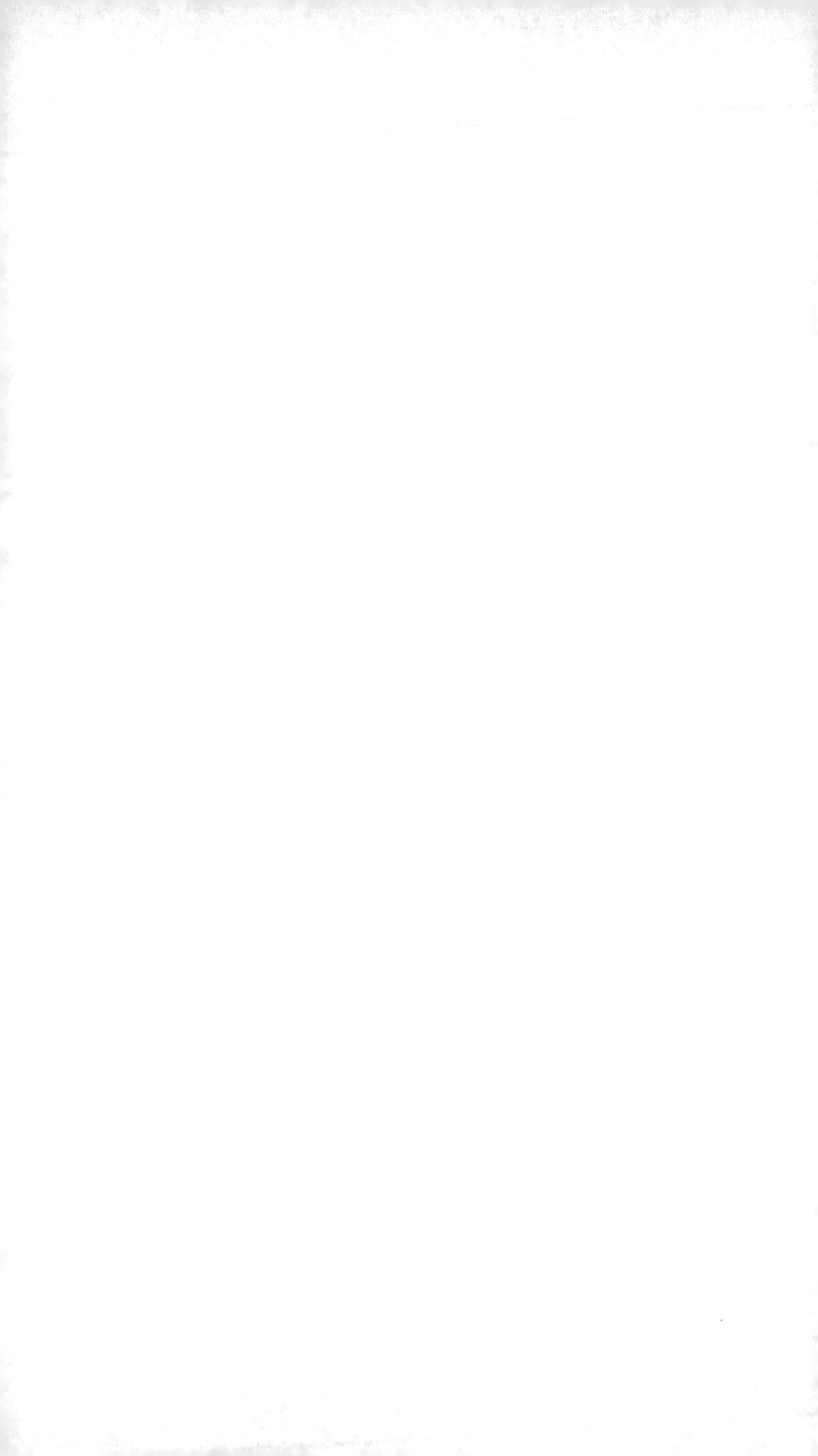

my greatest fear in life
is that it will all go by
without you in it.

should i tell them
that behind my smile there is a deep pain inside?

should i tell them
how i'm fighting back tears though my eyes are
open wide?

should i tell them
how i wait hopelessly and pray day and night?

should i tell them
or would opening my heart be a useless fight?

maybe i'll tell them
how their complaints and full arms look to me.

perhaps i'll tell them
that what they have is what i long to be.

it's been forever
since i thought of anything
except for you and the moon.

days in the sun
turn to years in the dark
all flashing by
as i wait for my tomorrow.

i'm searching for the happily ever after.
the chance to turn tears into laughter.
but when no one can tell me
why my body's a disaster
my mind goes numb
nothing else seems to matter.

how much longer
do you need to get here,
because time does not wait.
time does not pause
it does not stop
it does not look back for you
it does not rewind.
time does not wait.
no matter how many times i ask.

two more weeks
is all it'll be.

lap after lap
around the sun.
minutes and hours
pass one by one.

it's taken this long
for you to come home.
to be here with us,
no longer alone.

i've waited my entire life for this,
two more weeks won't kill me yet.

my eyes know not
what my soul gives to me.

my hands are yet to hold
what my heart can already see.

they tell me how this will go
they tell me how it should be
they tell me what medicine to take
but no one ever asks about me.

one by one they leave the room
with their words echoing down the hall
as i wait for my last grain of hope
i ask the universe for it all.

tell me why he's not here.
tell me why i feel so small.
tell me why it's happening to me.
tell me something, tell me anything at all.

there is no greater definition of irony
than wanting to give your entire heart to another
whose existence remains a mystery.

if love is enough to bring you home,
then you should be here any day now.

i'll wait for you
here in this chair
i'll count the days
until our time.
the tides will change
the sun will shine
days will come
and weeks go by
but my darling,
i will wait for you here.

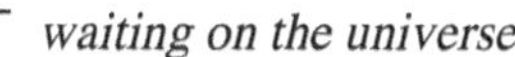

i would rather run a million miles into the sun
if it leads me straight to you
than to walk each and every day
aimlessly searching in the dark.

chapter two: loss

july 2014 - february 2015

Just when I was beginning to grasp the difficulty of conceiving a child, something miraculous happened. After countless fertility drugs, hormone injections, and four intrauterine inseminations (IUI), in the spring of 2014 the test came back positive. I was finally pregnant!

We cautiously walked into the exam room, quietly giggling inside jokes fueled by nerves and an unyielding fear of being told the test was wrong. The doctor turned on the camera and right there on the ultrasound screen was our baby. We were filled with joy and for the first time I found peace knowing that I indeed could get pregnant.

A few months later, on a hot day in July, I had a miscarriage. The night before I remember having a dream it was a baby boy. "He" was the size of an olive. I grimaced when people referred to the miscarriage as "losing the baby" implying that I misplaced it or did something wrong. I now know there was nothing I could have done differently. But on that day, a day that has replayed over and over in my mind, I felt guilt. I was pregnant for 10 weeks and 5 days. And then suddenly he was gone.

We said goodbye to the baby that was no longer growing. The baby I thought was meant to be and had hoped to hold someday. I felt the physical pain that came with miscarriage and the emotional weight of anger and disappointment at my body for once again failing me. My heart was broken and I was back at the start, wondering if or when I would ever become a mother.

she packed her bag
the one kept neatly
under her bed
with all the things
they said to bring.
they arrived
and as they waited
she took out the photo
the one kept proudly
in her wallet
admired so often
she could tell you
every detail of every
white blurry line.
they moved her bed
rolling her into
the next room
a sea of eyes looking
but not speaking
wearing gloves
and forced smiles
ready to play
their roles routinely.
the hardest day of her
life was just another
tuesday to them.

ten minutes later
the doctor arrived
he looked at the photo
but this time
no one smiled.
she packed her bag
this time to go home
they rode back
in silence
the bag on her lap
the ultrasound photo
wrinkled and tattered
from holding so tightly
in her hands
the only photo of him
she would ever have
but one she knew
so well
as small as an olive
with tiny arms
tiny feet
and a tiny heart
that she was told
only moments ago,
was no longer
beating.

on the day that he left,
the sun was shining for miles.
but i walked through the dark
displaced among a sea of smiles.

i took a deep breath.
i filled my body with air.
i felt a pain on my chest
knowing that he wasn't there.

i carried his breath,
for his was mine and mine was his.
my body was his home to grow
until one day it no longer was.

i took a deep breath.
i can still feel him here.
maybe tomorrow i'll exhale.
maybe tomorrow this will all feel real.

i wanted to love him forever
but he had other plans in mind.

i wanted to show him the world
but he decided some other time.

i wanted to kiss his sweet face
to see if it looked like his father's or mine.

but his image now lives for eternity
as only a daydream in the back of my mind.

i wanted those nine months of him
to carry him safely home.

but i guess that was too much to ask
and now i guess i'll never know.

just like that
he was gone.
gone like the daylight
ripped from the sun.
he never got to see its light
or feel its warmth upon his skin.
but he was never cold,
he was never alone,
and as long as i have love to give,
he will forever be ours.

tell the earth to stop turning,
for i can't bear another day without him here.
tell the birds there will be no more chirping,
for their songs are no longer music to my ear.

tell the sun to stop shining,
i have no use for its brightness in the sky.
and you can tell the rain to stop coming
there are enough drops from my own two eyes.

but if the world must go on spinning,
and a new day arrives without him here,
i'll think of him in another place
and softly smile knowing he is there.

in a place where the sun never sets,
where the flowers are always in bloom,
where he is alive and nothing is hurting him,
forever alive among the stars and the moon.

maybe some things
were never meant to be.
maybe he was never going
to find his way to me.

how could i have lost something
that was never mine to hold?

earthside would have been
a nice place to meet.
but he found somewhere else,
an entire universe at his feet.

as each month passes
i break more and more
shattered like glass
on the bathroom floor.
each time they try to fix me
gluing my pieces
to make me new.
but an impossible task
is becoming whole
when the missing piece
is always you.

he left me with an ocean full of tears,
but i learned long ago
how to sail towards the sun.

i painted a smile over all my scars
and fought back tears as big as the sea.
with a lump in my throat
i said i was fine.
i could fool almost anyone.
anyone,
          except for me.

"your sorrow,"

my love said to me,

"i'll carry as if it were mine."

and right there on the porch that night,

i knew i would never have to do this alone.

if this is the way it's supposed to be
then i'll see him in heaven.
don't wait up for me.

i often wonder who he would have been.
what kind of person he would turn out to be.

perhaps one day when my time has come
i will finally get the chance to see.

when i am sitting on a cloud up above
peacefully floating with nowhere to go

maybe then they'll bring me my baby.
maybe then i will finally know.

i'm sorry we never gave him a name
or heard how it sounded out loud.

we never saw the color of his eyes.
whether brown or blue like the sky.

his hands we'll never get to hold
but i loved him
and this i'll always know.

i wonder if one day
somewhere in my dreams
i'll find him among the stars.

"time heals,"
        they said to me one day.
but maybe that's not true.
maybe time just moves memories
to a different space in our hearts
making room for the new ones to join.

i no longer hide my tears
when my heart begins to ache.
for they remind me each time
that for a moment
i was wide awake.

no matter how long it lasted,
what a beautiful thing it is
to have had someone to love.

chapter three: hope

march 2015 - february 2016

I don't remember the exact moment my grieving ended. Perhaps a small part of me always will. But I do know that one day laughter starting to replace tears. And hope returned to our home.

We began meeting with new doctors to determine where to go from here. One doctor told me I needed to "make peace" with the fact that I may never get pregnant. Determined to prove them wrong, I let the optimistic side of me take over. I may not be very good at making babies, but turns out I am also not very good at "making peace."

We learned new words like *intracytoplasmic sperm injection* and *saline sonohysterogram*. And while adoption was always in the back of my mind, there was a part of me that longed to become pregnant. To watch my stomach grow; to feel kicks and heartbeats and hiccups inside of me that were not my own; and to see what it would be like to grow a human that looked like me and the man I loved. I wanted this. And more than anything I wanted to feel normal for wanting this.

We came up with a new plan and decided to try everything we could for one more chance to carry a child. In March of 2015 I started an aggressive dose of egg stimulating hormones in an attempt to get my body to release the few eggs that remained in my low ovarian reserves. It was the first step towards an in-vitro fertilization, also known as IVF. It was the most mentally, physically, and financially exhausting thing I have ever done. And knowing now how it turned out, I wouldn't change a single thing.

some sorrows are so deep
they take your breath away.
but it is only once you begin to seek joy
that you learn how to breathe again.

i'll tell you the story of a hero.
how he loved a girl
and she loved him back.
yet she needed to be rescued
time and time again.

when those moments arrived,
he wore no armed metal
no cape on his back
or badge of honor upon his chest.
for it wasn't physical strength that saved the day.

as he wiped away the tear
from the side of her cheek
as he had done so many times before,
she looked up and saw his eyes
filled with those very same tears.

our hero said nothing at all
and yet it was everything
she needed to hear.

the morning light is my favorite to see,
for it's one more day
bringing you closer to me.

sorrow never stays in one place for too long.
i welcomed it like a familiar house guest claiming
the best room. i gave it shelter and fed it a feast of
tears. i lay awake in bed listening to it crashing
and banging on the walls inside my head. but one
day it was gone, quietly slipping out the back
door. when i woke up i wondered if we'd see each
other again some day. for the rooms are now
filling up. hope is waiting at the door eager to be
checked in. and when hope comes around, she
always stays much longer.

out of all the memories i've ever made,
my favorite one is yet to come.

under the oaks
at the turn in the bend
there is a tiny home
that lies at the end of the street
surrounded by trees
taller than you've ever seen.
and through the kitchen
there's a room made up of only glass
where the sun pours in
through the branches
letting light flicker around
in a synchronized dance
that the sun has been practicing for years.
a little wooden rocking horse stands
motionless in the corner of the room
waiting for its opening act.
as i lie awake on the couch
my feet propped on the armrest
my eyes gazed out through the back door
the branches sway and whisper in the wind.
and it is then that i realize
these four walls are waiting
to welcome you home.

hope is holding onto something even when the rest of the world has let it go.

she's the one who dreams
with eyes wide open.
who hears the people
shouting for her to stop
but instead runs even further
towards the horizon.

she's the one who waits
for the universe to bring
the one meaningful thing
she'd give her life to find.

she's the one who dreams,
and won't stop
until the dream she sees each day
has finally come true.

they say there are plenty of fish in the sea,
but i'll wait for the tide to bring you here to me.

don't fight the tears from coming
for they will cleanse a broken heart
just as they always have
each and every time.

as that last teardrop hits the floor
you stand yourself back up and
find that you are stronger now.
stronger than you have ever been.
strong enough to fall in love again.

the most ordinary thing you can do
is to wish for the extraordinary.

sure the easy choice is to give up,
        i said to them one day.
but that's the thing about a mother's heart
        it will always fight back.

somewhere in between life
the drama
the hustle
the pain
and the sorrow
there is joy.
and because you have been through it all
when you finally do find joy
it will be greater
than you ever imagined.

you may have to wait a little longer.
your day will come.
your baby will arrive.
the sun is shining for you.
and there is light headed your way.

the world is full of beautiful miracles.
maybe one of them was meant for me.

a *maybe baby*
were the words
when there was nothing left to say.
a *someday baby*
brings me hope
for my someday is on its way.

tomorrow seems like a good place to be.
i'll see you there,
when the sun meets the sea.

storms will rage
and then they pass.
the clouds will finally let go.

the sun will awaken
again in the sky
and there we'll see our rainbow.

if i knew then
what i know now,
i'd still do it all over again.
i'd make an ocean's worth of tears
waiting for you.
i'd toss thousands of dollars
into a barrel
and watch it drift away with the tide.
i now know it all happened
just as it was supposed to.
exactly how it happened,
to lead you here to me.

i pray that life surprises you one day.
your jaw drops to the floor
with no words left to say.

for what they told you
couldn't possibly be,
instead is now a miracle
timed imperfectly.

but if it turns out
things don't go that route
i hope you'll keep shining
and storming about.

for that's the thing
about every new day,
there's plenty more
that are on their way.

whenever you feel like hope is gone,
take a deep breath
and remember some miracles
are just moments away.

succeeding
feels like the hardest thing to do,
but to love ourselves
even when we fail,
that is the most difficult
yet significant thing
you'll ever achieve.

it's easy to lose hope
but even easier to find it again
especially if you know where to look.
hope is in the sunshine
that hits your window each morning
welcoming a new day.
hope can be found resting
in the palm of someone's hand,
reaching out to be comforted by your warmth.
hope is in the very air that you breathe,
it's in the clouds
and it's in the rain,
giving this same planet that you stand upon,
another chance to turn things around.
and on that cobblestone street
in charleston that day,
as we paced back and forth,
watching the minutes
slowly tick by
and waiting under a hot humid sky,
we discovered
that hope found its way back to us once again.

and right there,
that one part of my heart
next to the spot
where grief lived for so many years,
is now slowly being filled,
by the love of a baby boy.
as if it had always been there
simply tucked away
hidden behind the shadows of sorrow,
just waiting for its time to shine.

you're here.
it's you.
it's always been you.
and as our eyes meet for the very first time
my soul finally sighed.
relief.
peace.
undeniable joy.
knowing how long
i waited on the universe
to bring me you.
and now you're here.
it's you i was waiting for, my darling.
it's always been you.

about the author

Priscilla Brown is a writer, a dreamer, a hopeful world traveler, a speech pathologist, a wife, and a mother. She is passionate about speaking out and supporting other couples going through infertility. *waiting on the universe* is her first book of poetry. She currently lives in Charleston, South Carolina in a house with a garden with her husband and their two sons who were both IVF babies and both born on February 14, exactly three years apart.

special thanks

I would like to give a special thanks to Will, the moon that holds our universe together. Whether it is books or babies, thank you for always believing in my dreams.

To my family and friends, thank you for your always present, everlasting love.

To my editor and to Celena, thank you for helping turn my pile of words into an actual book.

Thank you to anyone in the infertility community, your hope and determination continues to inspire me daily.

And thank you so very much to my readers for your support. I hope you'll stick around for what's coming next!

stay connected

join Priscilla online at

priscillatbrown.com